# Getting Your Cycle Back On Track: Reclaiming Your Fertility and Hormonal Health

**Getting Your Cycle Back On Track: Reclaiming Your Fertility and Hormonal Health**

# Table of Content

# Introduction

Having a healthy, regular menstrual cycle is an important sign that your body is functioning as it should. But amidst the busyness of modern life, many women experience absent, irregular, or painful periods without understanding why. Skipped cycles or unpredictable bleeding can negatively impact your fertility, health, and quality of life.

If you've noticed your normal rhythms are off, you're not alone. Abnormal periods affect approximately one in five women. Causes range from hormonal imbalances and ovarian problems to high stress levels, nutritional deficiencies, and underlying medical conditions. When periods go MIA for months on end, it's known as amenorrhea.

The absence of a monthly cycle is your body's way of communicating that something is out of balance. But with the right support and guidance, you can get your cycle back on track and reclaim your hormonal health. This book will be your comprehensive guide to understanding irregular menstruation, identifying potential causes, and learning natural and medical solutions to restore your fertility.

Inside, you'll find science-based and holistic strategies to:

- Better understand the intricate hormonal dance underlying the phases of your menstrual cycle.

- Pinpoint possible reasons for missed or irregular periods specific to your symptoms and history.

- Make lifestyle changes to reduce stress, improve your diet, optimize sleep, balance hormones, and encourage a healthy cycle.

- Utilize herbal supplements and natural therapies to support your reproductive system.

- Know when to seek medical testing and treatment for underlying issues.

- Take charge of your fertility and maximize your chances of conception.

You'll also find compassionate support and a judgment-free approach. Your periods hold unique insights about your personal health. By learning to decode the messages of your body, you can address issues early and prevent long-term complications. Consider this book your resource to work alongside practitioners and advocate for your own wellbeing.

Regaining your cycles requires patience and self-care. But with the tools in this book, you'll gain confidence to eliminate period problems, improve hormone balance, and create a fertile foundation. Healthy monthly rhythms are within your reach.

Let's get started decoding your body's signals, solving cycle mysteries, and putting your menstrual health back into your own hands. With consistency and time, you can get your cycle back on track.

# Chapter 1: Understanding Your Menstrual Cycle

Your menstrual cycle is an intricate hormonal symphony conducted each month to prepare your body for potential pregnancy. When functioning normally, this cyclic rise and fall of hormones regulates menstrual bleeding and promotes ovulation.

Understanding the distinct fertility phases and fluctuations of hormones throughout your cycle empowers you to identify abnormalities, trace symptoms to their source, and regain balance. In this foundational chapter, we'll explore:

- The four menstrual phases and their hormone patterns

- What defines a normal cycle?

- When irregularities become problematic

- How to track your cycles

- Ways to work with your natural rhythms

## The Menstrual Phase

The first phase of each cycle begins on day one of your period, when the shedding of your uterine lining causes bleeding to start. Estrogen and progesterone levels are low at this time, triggering the uterus to contract and slough off tissue that accumulated during the previous cycle.

The drop in estrogen and progesterone signals your pituitary gland to ramp up production of follicle stimulating hormone (FSH) and luteinizing hormone (LH). These hormones initiate the recruitment of immature ovarian follicles to begin developing.

During this phase, which lasts about five days on average, you'll experience menstrual flow ranging from light to heavy. Common symptoms include:

- Cramps and pain as the uterus contracts
- Fatigue
- Bloating
- Lower back pain
- Headaches
- Food cravings
- Mood changes and irritability

Your flow usually transitions from bright red to dark brown or pink as the phase winds down. Bleeding stops when estrogen levels begin rising again.

# The Follicular Phase

As blood estrogen slowly increases in the follicular phase, the pituitary gland releases more FSH, which stimulates a cohort of follicles to mature. One dominant follicle typically emerges about seven days before ovulation.

Inside this lead follicle, an egg starts developing while the follicle itself produces more estrogen. This rising estrogen thickens the uterine lining and cervical mucus. The switch from your menstrual flow to creamy cervical fluid marks the beginning of the follicular phase.

Lasting between 10-22 days, this phase encompasses:

- Recruitment of follicles
- Selection of the dominant follicle
- Maturation of an egg cell

- Growth of the endometrium

- Increased cervical mucus

The length of the follicular phase determines the total length of your cycle. Longer phases indicate delayed ovulation. A short follicular phase may prevent the uterine lining from adequately thickening before an egg is released.

# The Ovulatory Phase

In the middle of your cycle, 24-36 hours before your egg emerges, estrogen peaks triggering a surge of LH from the pituitary gland. This LH surge kickstarts the process of ovulation.

As ovulation approaches, cervical fluid becomes wet, stretchy, and slippery–resembling raw egg whites. This fluid fosters sperm motility. Your basal body temperature also drops slightly just before the LH peak.

During ovulation, which lasts about 24-48 hours, the dominant follicle ruptures and releases its mature egg into the Fallopian tube. The remnants of the follicle transform into the corpus luteum, which starts secreting progesterone and estrogen.

Physical cues of ovulation include:

- Stretchy, egg white-like cervical fluid

- Abdominal cramps or twinges

- Increased libido

- Breast tenderness

- Light spotting

Ovulation predictor kits detect the pre-ovulatory LH surge in urine about 12-36 hours before ovulation. Tracking basal body temperature identifies the post-ovulatory temperature spike.

# The Luteal Phase

After ovulation, progesterone production from the corpus luteum prepares the uterus to implant a fertilized egg. Estrogen levels also remain elevated.

Lasting 12-16 days, the luteal phase includes:

- Continued follicle remnant secretion

- Lining of uterus becomes spongy

- Cervical mucus thickens

If an egg is fertilized, the embryo will implant 6-12 days after ovulation. The corpus luteum continues producing hormones to support the pregnancy.

Without fertilization, the corpus luteum degenerates causing sharp declines in estrogen and progesterone. This triggers menstruation and your next cycle.

Short luteal phases under 10 days can make implantation difficult. Low progesterone hampers adequate endometrial thickening.

Symptoms in the luteal phase stem from elevated hormones and premenstrual syndrome (PMS). Fatigue, mood changes, breast tenderness, bloating, and cramps are common.

# What's Considered Normal?

Menstrual cycle lengths are quite varied, but a cycle between 21-35 days is deemed normal and healthy. Duration from the first day of one period to the next averages 28 days.

Ovulation typically occurs close to the midpoint of your cycle. So in a 28 day cycle, ovulation happens around day 14. But the timing of ovulation determines the length of each phase:

**Follicular Phase:** Can range from 10 to 22 days

**Ovulation:** Lasts 24 to 48 hours

**Luteal Phase:** Ranges from 10 to 16 days

Regular cycles indicate your endocrine system is functioning properly. Getting familiar with your personal menstrual patterns makes it easier to identify irregularities.

# When Variability Becomes Problematic

While some fluctuations in cycle length are normal, excessive variability or patterns of very long/short cycles can signify issues including:

- Impaired ovulation

- Hormone imbalances

- Ovarian dysfunction

- Endometriosis

- Structural problems

- High stress

- Thyroid disorders

- PCOS

- Premature ovarian failure

Absent periods for over 3 months is termed amenorrhea. This often results from:

- Pregnancy

- Breastfeeding

- Menopause

- Eating disorders

- Excessive exercise

- PCOS

- Premature ovarian failure

- Medical conditions

If you miss periods or experience sudden unexplained changes in your cycle, see your doctor to uncover potential causes. Track your cycles to pinpoint patterns.

# Get Familiar with Your Cycles

Understanding when you ovulate and when to expect your period gives you greater body awareness. Consider tracking key fertility signs:

- **Record cycle lengths:** Document the first day of each menstrual cycle so you can identify when your period becomes irregular.

- **Check cervical fluid:** Fluid changes throughout your cycle offer clues into your most fertile days.

- **Monitor basal body temperature:** A basal thermometer detects the slight dip and spike surrounding ovulation.

- **Use ovulation predictor kits:** These detect impending ovulation by measuring LH levels in urine.

- **Track symptoms:** Record how you feel each day to make connections.

- **Note sexual activity:** Together with cycle data, this timing may indicate pregnancy.

Apps, journals, and fertility charts help compile the data into insights about your hormonal patterns. Share tracking with your doctor.

# Working with Your Cycles

Cooperating with your natural rhythms can enhance your menstrual health:

- Support each phase with nutrition and lifestyle.

- Avoid toxic exposures from plastics and chemicals that disrupt hormones.

- Reduce stress and anxiety which impair reproductive function.

- Get sufficient sleep, exercise, and relaxation. Balance your workload.

- Ride the energy waves of each phase and adjust activities accordingly.

- Time demanding tasks for after menstruation and before ovulation.

Now that you better comprehend the intricacies of your monthly cycle, you can identify your body's signs of distress and implement solutions to restore hormonal harmony. Robust menstrual health equates to overall wellbeing.

# Chapter 2: Common Causes of Absent or Irregular Periods

If your cycles have gone awry, pinpointing the underlying cause is key to getting your rhythm back. Abnormal periods result from disruptions anywhere along the hormonal pathway of the hypothalamic-pituitary-ovarian axis.

In this chapter, we'll explore the wide range of potential reasons for missing or irregular menstrual cycles, including:

- Hormonal imbalances

- Ovarian issues

- Ovulation problems

- Endocrine disorders

- Uterine abnormalities

- Excessive weight loss

- Eating disorders

- Extreme exercise

- High stress

- Medications

- Chronic medical conditions

- Perimenopause

Understanding common culprits behind irregular menstruation allows you to track symptoms, advocate for proper testing, and find tailored solutions.

## Fluctuating Hormones

The meticulous dance of hormones along the HPO axis determines the timing and flow of your period. Imbalances in estrogen, progesterone, FSH, LH and other hormones often underlie cycle irregularities:

**High estrogen levels** can halt ovulation and cause breakthrough mid-cycle spotting. Sources include obesity, tumors, and estrogen dominance.

**Low estrogen** prevents adequate endometrial thickening for menstruation. Causes include low body weight, high stress, thyroid disorder, and premature ovarian failure.

**Progesterone deficiency** in the luteal phase makes it harder for a fertilized egg to implant. This leads to shorter cycles.

**High androgens**, like testosterone, contribute to missed ovulation. Women with PCOS often have elevated androgens.

**High prolactin** from tumors and medications inhibits proper LH and FSH signaling.

Testing hormone levels can identify imbalances. Targeted treatments like supplements or medication can often restore optimal balances.

# Ovarian Dysfunction

As the site of egg maturation and ovulation, our ovaries are pivotal to menstrual health. Ovarian problems like these can lead to irregular or absent cycles:

**Polycystic Ovary Syndrome (PCOS):** Characterized by multiple cysts, high androgens, absent/irregular periods, and ovulation issues. Caused by insulin resistance.

**Premature Ovarian Failure (POF):** Menopause before age 40 due to depleted ovaries. Usually leads to irregular cycles then cessation.

**Ovarian Insufficiency:** Reduced ovarian function due to cancer treatment, autoimmune disease, genetics, or unknown cause.

**Ovarian Cysts:** Fluid-filled sacs which can develop on ovaries and impact hormone production and ovulation.

**Endometriosis:** When uterine tissue grows outside uterus often affecting ovaries. Can distort pelvic anatomy.

Treatment focuses on addressing the underlying ovarian issue through medication, diet changes or sometimes surgery.

# Ovulation Issues

Since ovulation kickstarts the next cycle phase, absent or impaired ovulation disrupts menstrual rhythms. What inhibits ovulation?

- High stress
- Being over- or underweight
- Hormone imbalances
- Ovarian problems like PCOS
- Thyroid disorders
- Damage to ovaries
- Pelvic inflammation
- Endometriosis

Signs of ovulation issues:

- Irregular cycle lengths
- Lack of ovulation pain/cramping
- Absence of fertile cervical fluid
- No premenstrual symptoms
- High LH but no LH surge

Tracking ovulation with BBT charts or urine tests can confirm suspected ovulation problems. Ovulation induction medications like Clomid might be used short-term to spur ovulation.

# Endocrine System Disorders

The endocrine network of glands and hormones are intrinsically tied to menstrual cycle regulation. Endocrine disorders can commonly cause irregular cycles:

**Thyroid problems** like hypothyroidism, hyperthyroidism, and autoimmune thyroid disease impact cycle length and fertility.

**Elevated prolactin** from tumors, medicines, or unknown causes inhibits LH/FSH preventing ovulation.

**Adrenal issues** producing excess cortisol can suppress ovulation and sex hormones.

**Diabetes** causes hormone fluctuations that affect ovulation and cycle regularity.

**Pituitary tumors** overproducing prolactin, or underproducing LH/FSH, interfere with normal cycles.

Testing thyroid, glucose, and hormone levels identifies endocrine problems. Addressing the root disorder or using medications to regulate endocrine function may restore normal cycles.

# Uterine Abnormalities

Structural or anatomical disorders of the uterus can also contribute to painful, heavy, irregular, or missed periods:

- **Fibroids:** Benign muscle tumors which can distort uterine shape and cavity.

- **Polyps:** Overgrowths of endometrial tissue that protrude into the uterus.

- **Adenomyosis:** When endometrial tissue grows into the uterine muscle walls.

- **Uterine scarring:** From procedures like dilation and curettage (D&C).

- **Congenital anomalies:** Such as a septate or bicornuate uterus.

- **Asherman's syndrome:** Scarring within the uterine cavity due to infection or surgery.

Depending on the abnormality, treatment may include surgical removal, hormone therapy, or IVF.

# Weight Loss and Eating Disorders

Dramatic decreases in body weight disrupt ovulation and throw off menstrual cycles:

- Losing >10% body weight through dieting, digestive issues, overexercise or eating disorders often causes amenorrhea.

- Extreme caloric restriction inhibits production of leptin from fat cells. Low leptin impairs GnRH release stalling reproductive hormones.

- Rapid fat loss stresses the HPO axis. Energy deficiency signals the body to halt non-essential functions like ovulation.

- Once BMI drops below 18.5, periods often stop and don't resume until normal weight is restored.

- Anorexia, bulimia, binge eating disorder and OSFED also commonly cause abnormal periods.

Healing nutrition that restores weight and caloric intake will help bring back menstrual cycles. Ovulation and regular rhythms typically resume once weight normalizes.

# The Exercise Connection

Alongside low BMI, excessive exercise also disrupts cycles by lowering leptin and body fat levels. Without adequate fuel stores, the hypothalamus suppresses reproductive function.

- Training more than 5 hours daily, or burning over 1000 calories from exercise, is linked to amenorrhea in female athletes and dancers.

- High-intensity, chronic cardio and burst training are more likely to impair cycles than moderate strength training.

- Up to 60% of elite dancers and female athletes experience menstrual dysfunction due to low energy availability.

- Effects are often reversible by reducing exercise volume, limiting intensity, and increasing caloric intake.

Balancing activity with reduced training, nutrition, and rest days allows the HPO axis to recover and restart cycles.

# The Stress Impact

Our menstrual cycle is very sensitive to perceptions of stress in the mind and environment. Stress triggers cortisol release which inhibits GnRH production, LH/FSH levels, ovulation, and menstruation.

- Emotional distress from relationships, work, finances, trauma, grief and anxiety often causes period problems.

- Women with depression have a higher likelihood of amenorrhea.

- Times of intense worry, pressure, and overwhelm commonly delay or disrupt cycles.

- Cortisol suppresses estrogen, gonadotropins, and progesterone secretion stalling reproductive function.

- Stress management through therapy, meditation, time-off, and self-care can help normalize cycles.

Bringing your nervous system back into balance reduces cortisol. This allows normal hormonal rhythms to resume.

# Medications and Contraceptives

Numerous pharmaceutical drugs directly impact the menstrual cycle leading to alterations in flow and timing:

- Hormonal contraceptives like the pill prevent ovulation leading to lighter withdrawal bleeding rather than a natural period.

- Antidepressants, antipsychotics, opioids, anticonvulsants and cytotoxic drugs change hormone levels which commonly causes irregular spotting.

- Corticosteroids and anxiety medications increase prolactin production preventing LH surge and ovulation.

- NSAIDs, blood thinners, chemotherapy, tranquilizers and ulcer medications can cause abnormal bleeding.

- Post-pill amenorrhea is common as the HPO axis recalibrates after stopping oral contraceptives.

Discuss medication effects with your prescriber. Adjusting dosages or switching drug types can often minimize cycle side effects.

# Medical Conditions

Various chronic illnesses and their treatments indirectly disturb menstrual cycles through effects on hormones, metabolism, inflammation and energy levels:

**Autoimmune diseases** like lupus, rheumatoid arthritis, and multiple sclerosis often impair menstrual regularity and ovulation.

**Gastrointestinal diseases** including Crohn's, ulcerative colitis, and celiac disease impact nutrient absorption needed to sustain cycles.

**Heart and lung diseases** reduce oxygen circulation necessary for reproductive organ function.

**Diabetes** causes hormone and insulin fluctuations which hinder ovulation.

**Kidney disease** leads to hormonal imbalances that commonly cause absent periods.

**Cancer** and chemotherapy damage the ovaries accelerating menopause and cycle changes.

**HIV** causes immunological effects and nutritional deficits that can shift hormone levels and disrupt periods.

Successfully managing the primary medical condition may help minimize impacts on menstruation. But additional reproductive treatment is often needed.

# Perimenopause

As ovarian function starts declining in your 30s and 40s, the transition to menopause causes highly irregular cycles and ovulation changes:

- Cycle length often varies widely during perimenopause which spans several years before menopause.

- You might skip periods for months then have heavy flow the next cycle.

- Estrogen levels rise and fall unevenly leading to more breakthrough bleeding.

- Failed ovulation results in more common anovulatory cycles without a true period.

- Luteal phase shortens due to dropping progesterone as egg quality declines.

- FSH readings start to increase as your ovaries respond less efficiently.

- Premenstrual symptoms often worsen.

Abnormal cycles during the menopausal transition are normal. But sudden onset requires ruling out benign abnormalities like fibroids or polyps.

Pinpointing what's amiss internally empowers you to find solutions. Tracking symptoms against your cycle can identify hormonal connections. Work with your doctor to diagnose the cause, implement targeted treatments, and restore your rhythmic flow.

# Chapter 3: Lifestyle Changes That Support Healthy Cycles

The right lifestyle habits create an environment in your body that allows your menstrual cycle to thrive. Small daily choices to reduce stress, exercise moderately, support hormonal balance through nutrition, minimize toxins, and get adequate rest all profoundly influence the regulation of your monthly rhythm.

In this chapter, we'll explore practical lifestyle changes within your control that can get your cycles back on track:

- Managing stress and anxiety
- Optimizing sleep
- Balancing exercise
- Eliminating toxic exposures
- Improving your diet
- Supporting healthy body weight
- Reducing alcohol intake
- Quitting smoking

## Stress Management Strategies

Perceived stress elicits the fight-or-flight response which triggers cortisol release. Cortisol suppresses the hypothalamic secretion of GnRH stalling reproductive hormones and ovulation.

To counteract stress:

**Cultivate daily relaxation** through deep breathing, meditation, visualization, nature time and calming activities. Make leisure and fun a priority.

**Try talk therapy** to process emotions, trauma, and relationship dynamics that contribute to anxiety.

**Improve time management** and organization to prevent overwhelm. Set realistic deadlines and delegate tasks.

**Identify and modify stress triggers** related to work, finances, family, health or other causes of worry. Seek solutions.

**Learn to say no** and set boundaries around responsibilities. Don't overcommit yourself.

**Spend time with supportive people** who enrich your life and make you feel cared for.

**Take a stress-reducing vacation** or staycation to recharge. Disconnect from technology and obligations that drain you.

**Consider antidepressant or anti-anxiety medications** if anxiety is severe. But be cautious of associated menstrual side effects.

**Get assessed for cortisol levels** with saliva testing. High cortisol contributes to amenorrhea.

Dialing down stress helps rebalance hormones, sustain ovulation, and regulate your cycle.

# Prioritize Restorative Sleep

Alongside stress, lack of sufficient high-quality sleep disrupts hormonal pathways. Strive for:

- 7-9 hours nightly
- Consistent bedtime and wake-up time to sync circadian rhythm
- Limiting blue light exposure before bedtime
- Creating an optimal sleep environment that is cool, dark and quiet

- Avoidingstimulants like caffeine, alcohol, or heavy foods before bed

- Managing worries and racing thoughts using journaling or meditation before bed

- Skipping screens and digital stimulation for 1-2 hours pre-sleep

- Establishing a relaxing pre-bedtime routine

- Catching up on sleep debt using naps and weekends

Quality sleep allows reproductive hormones to follow natural rhythms needed for ovulation and regular cycles.

# Find Your Optimal Exercise Balance

Moderate exercise boosts energy, mood, and cardiovascular health which supports menstrual cycle regulation. But too much high-intensity exercise stresses the body, lowering BMI and body fat percentage. This suppresses reproductive function in favor of more essential biological processes.

Aim for:

- 150 minutes per week of moderate aerobic activity like brisk walking, swimming, hiking or gentle cycling

- 2-3 days per week of muscle-strengthening moves using resistance bands, weights or bodyweight

- Taking 1-2 rest days between intense workouts

- Avoiding excessive cardio like daily long runs which can impair ovulation

- Considering taking the first part of your cycle off from strenuous exercise

- Ensuring adequate calorie intake to fuel activity and maintain healthy BMI

- Increasing calories further if you experience amenorrhea

- Seeing a sports medicine doctor if you're exercising extensively with irregular periods

With a balanced workout routine guided by your body's cues, you can stay active without compromising your cycles.

# Eliminate Endocrine Disruptors

Toxins and chemicals called endocrine disruptors interfere with hormone pathways in the body contributing to irregular periods. Reduce exposure to:

**Plastics:** Especially BPA and phthalates that leach from food containers, water bottles, toys, beauty products and PVC pipes. Use glass or stainless steel instead.

**Conventional personal care items:** Containing parabens, formaldehyde, triclosan, and xylene. Opt for organic, green brands.

**Pesticides, herbicides, fungicides:** Found on non-organic produce, cotton and grains. Eat organic when possible and wash produce.

**Growth hormones and antibiotics:** Given to conventionally raised meat and dairy animals. Choose organic grass-fed options.

**Gasoline, diesel exhaust, industrial chemicals:** Avoid breathing in fumes when possible. Filter indoor air.

**Heating food or drinks in plastic:** Never microwave in plastic. Don't pour hot liquid into Styrofoam or lined cups.

The fewer hormone disruptors your body absorbs, the more likely your endocrine system can maintain its delicate balance.

# Adopt a Menstrual-Friendly Diet

Nutrition lays the foundation for hormonal health. Follow these diet tips:

**Get sufficient calories** to fuel ovulatory cycles yet avoid weight gain. Moderate caloric restriction or restrictive diets lead to low leptin levels, metabolic stress, and amenorrhea.

**Minimize processed foods, sugar and refined grains:** These spike blood sugar causing insulin resistance and inflammation shown to block ovulation.

**Eat plant-based organic whole foods:** Vegetables, fruits, beans, lentils, whole grains supply antioxidants and phytonutrients that balance hormones.

**Choose healthy fats:** Omega-3s and monounsaturated fats improve insulin sensitivity for optimal hormone signaling.

**Reduce conventional meat and dairy:** Conventionally raised animals ingest hormones and antibiotics that can impact cycles when consumed. Choose organic and grass-fed.

**Eat fermented foods daily:** Sauerkraut, kimchi, kefir, yogurt, kombucha support digestive and vaginal microbiome balance to remove excess estrogen from the body.

**Stay hydrated:** Meet your daily water needs to aid liver detoxification.

**Limit alcohol and caffeine:** Both stimulate the adrenals causing hormone fluctuations. Restrict to 1-2 servings daily max.

A whole food, fiber-rich, anti-inflammatory diet resets hormones for cycle regularity.

# Achieve a Healthy Weight

Maintaining a BMI within the healthy range has an enormous influence on menstrual health. Too little body fat suppresses reproductive hormones triggering amenorrhea. Excess body fat boosts estrogen and inflammatory cytokines that hinder ovulation.

Aim for a BMI between 20-25:

- If underweight with a BMI below 18, put on some pounds through weightlifting and increased calorie intake. Fullness cues from leptin are needed to switch the HPO axis back on.

- If overweight with a BMI above 25, adopt a balanced hypocaloric diet and gradual consistent exercise routine. Losing just 5% excess body weight can jumpstart ovulation.

- Calorie restrict mindfully, avoiding deficits above 500 daily to prevent metabolic stress. Higher deficits shock the system.

- Focus on sustainable lifestyle change, not short-term fad diets which backfire long-term.

Your body functions optimally within a healthy weight range that supports ovulation and hormonal harmony.

# Limit Alcohol Intake

Alcohol disrupts hormone balance via multiple mechanisms:

- Suppresses FSH needed for proper follicular development

- Impacts ovulation timing and luteal phase progesterone levels

- Causes estrogen levels to spike outside the fertile window

- Increases risk of luteal phase spotting and bleeding

- Chronic drinking exacerbates insulin resistance and inflammation

- Contributes to weight gain and increased belly fat influencing estrogen

- Stresses the liver compromising its role detoxifying excess hormones

Restrict intake to no more than 1-2 servings daily. Avoid binge drinking episodes which can significantly disrupt your cycle that month.

# Quit Smoking

The toxins in cigarette smoke compromise female fertility and menstrual cycle health:

- Mutates DNA inside ovaries accelerating depletion

- Impairs folliculogenesis and embryo implantation

- Lowers estrogen levels needed for uterine lining development

- Causes earlier menopause onset

- Linked to luteal phase defects

- Compounds infertility issues

Quitting improves hormonal balance, ovarian reserve, egg quality, and menstrual regularity.

---

Restructuring your daily habits and environment to be more cycle-friendly helps restore your natural rhythms. With consistent nurturing lifestyle changes, you create the optimal backdrop against which your menstrual cycle can thrive.

# Chapter 4: Herbal and Natural Therapies

Alongside lifestyle measures, certain herbal supplements, essential oils, Traditional Chinese Medicine, and Ayurveda offer time-tested natural solutions to address hormonal imbalances underlying irregular periods.

In this chapter, we'll explore holistic therapies that can be used safely alongside medical treatment to restore cycle regularity:

- Targeted herbs and supplements

- Essential oils for hormonal support

- Traditional Chinese Medicine

- Acupuncture

- Ayurvedic therapies

Always consult your healthcare provider before starting new herbal supplements and natural remedies. Stop using if any allergic reactions or side effects occur.

## Herbs and Supplements for Hormonal Balance

Herbs and certain nutritional supplements can gently re-balance your reproductive hormones for improved cycle regulation:

**Chasteberry (Vitex):** Regulates LH and FSH to stimulate ovulation. Also increases progesterone. Helpful for PCOS.

**Black Cohosh:** Alleviates estrogen dominance by occupying estrogen receptors. Used for irregular periods.

**Maca root:** Supports hormonal balance. Can help induce menstruation in amenorrhea.

**Dong quai:** Considered a "female ginseng". Regulates menstrual cycle timing. Helpful for irregular bleeding.

**Turmeric:** Has anti-inflammatory effects that improve insulin resistance related to ovarian cysts and hormone dysfunction.

**Omega-3 fatty acids:** Help optimize progesterone and estrogen levels. Corrects luteal phase defects.

**Vitamin C:** Improves progesterone levels in luteal phase. Lengthens the follicular phase to enable ovulation.

**Magnesium:** Deficiency contributes to low progesterone and estrogen imbalance. Supplementation aids regulation.

**Vitamin B6:** Part of the synthesis pathway of estrogen and progesterone. Supports overall hormonal balance.

**Evening primrose oil:** Provides building blocks for estrogen and prostaglandins. Traditionally used for PMS.

Herbs should be taken for several months to realize benefits. Effects are gradual but sustained. Always follow dosage guidelines.

# Essential Oils for Menstrual Support

Certain essential oils help modulate estrogen, improve mood issues related to cycle fluctuations, and relieve period cramps:

**Clary sage:** Has phytoestrogenic compounds that help regulate estrogen levels. Provides menstrual cramp relief.

**Rose:** Emotionally uplifting and calming. Helps reduce moodiness, anxiety and depression during menstruation.

**Ylang ylang:** An anti-inflammatory that also improves low moods and worries exacerbated premenstrually.

**Lavender:** Soothes the nervous system, assisting with PMS irritability and emotional sensitivity. Also eases menstrual cramps.

**Marjoram:** Anti-spasmodic action relieves uterine contractions, calms muscle tension and eases painful cramps.

Use a few drops in a warm bath, diffuse aromatically, massage diluted oils on the abdomen, or use in homemade lotion to rub on your lower belly.

# Traditional Chinese Medicine

This ancient system aims to restore balance within the body's energetic meridians and organs using herbs, acupuncture, dietary therapy, massage techniques and exercise:

**Acupuncture:** Releases endorphins which influence the hypothalamic-pituitary-ovarian pathway. Also improves blood flow to reproductive organs.

**Herbal formulas:** Custom combinations of herbs based on each woman's unique presentation to harmonize the menstrual cycle.

**Nutrition:** Dietary advice eliminates inflammatory foods that create hormone imbalance while emphasizing blood-nourishing foods.

**Abdominal massage:** Promotes Qi flow to uterus and ovaries to reduce pain, cramps, and stagnation.

**Qigong exercises:** These flowing movements enhance overall energy circulation throughout the body.

Chinese medicine offers a holistic toolkit to realign your hormonal environment, remove blockages, and restore your natural rhythms.

# Restoring Flow with Acupuncture

Acupuncture adjusts bodily systems by stimulating certain acupressure points using fine needles. This traditional therapy improves many menstrual irregularities:

- Regulates hormones creating a more ideal balance

- Corrects absent ovulation allowing menstruation to resume

- Reduces menstrual cramps and PMS discomfort

- Lessens heavy prolonged bleeding

- Helps with amenorrhea recovery and post-birth control pill amenorrhea

- Improves menstrual migraines and endometriosis pain

- Enhances fertility when trying to conceive

For best results, plan weekly treatments for at least 3 consecutive menstrual cycles along with herbal formulas prescribed by the acupuncturist based on your pattern diagnosis.

# Ayurvedic Approaches

This traditional Indian system aims to balance the three doshas which govern all bodily processes. Specific therapies normalize menstrual rhythms:

**Herbs and supplements:** Ayurveda utilizes many herbs to regulate hormones and promote ovulation like shatavari and ashwagandha.

**Abhyanga massage:** With dosha-specific herbal oils to improve circulation and relieve pain.

**Meditation:** Reduces cortisol and emotional distress which impair hormonal balance.

**Panchakarma detox:** Eliminates ama toxins through the cleansing action of herbs, massage, steam therapy, and laxatives.

**Dietary changes:** Emphasize fresh vegetables, fruits, legumes, whole grains and healthy fats tailored to your constitution.

Ayurveda's multifaceted therapies reduce systemic inflammation and stagnation for fuller, more regular flow.

Integrating natural solutions alongside medical treatments provides a comprehensive approach to realign your hormones and menstrual cycle. Herbs, supplements, essential oils, acupuncture, massage techniques, dietary changes, and stress reduction work synergistically to create optimal circumstances for regulation of your natural rhythms.

# Chapter 5: When to Seek Medical Help

If you've made lifestyle changes and tried natural therapies without resolving abnormal cycles, consulting a doctor for further evaluation is wise.

Medical testing can identify any underlying conditions contributing to your irregular menstruation so proper treatment can be implemented.

In this chapter, we'll cover:

- Working with your doctor

- Important medical tests

- Potential treatment options

- Medications that regulate periods

- When to consider IVF

Keep advocating for your health until you get to the root cause and find an effective solution.

## Partnering with Your Doctor

Describe your menstrual history and any changes you've observed to your physician. Keeping detailed records of your cycles, including:

- Cycle length

- Flow amount

- Pain

- Premenstrual symptoms

- Side effects

- Energy levels

- Sexual activity

- Ovulation predictors

- Basal body temperature

Armed with this data, your doctor can make informed choices about testing and next steps. If your concerns aren't taken seriously, seek a second opinion. A reproductive endocrinologist has specialized expertise. Questions to ask include:

- What might be causing my irregular cycles?

- Which tests do you recommend and why?

- What treatments are best for my situation?

- What side effects or risks are involved?

- Will treatment restore fertility if desired?

- How will we monitor progress?

- Are there any lifestyle changes that could also help?

Working collaboratively leads to solutions tailored to your circumstances.

# Diagnostic Testing

Based on your history and symptoms, your doctor will suggest tests to pinpoint causes. Common assessments include:

- **Blood hormone panel:** Measuring FSH, LH, estrogen, testosterone, DHEA-S, TSH for imbalances. Serum AMH also reflects ovarian reserve.

- **Transvaginal ultrasound:** Evaluates ovarian health and follicle count. Checks uterine structure.

- **HSG:** X-ray with dye that screens for uterine abnormalities like fibroids or polyps. Checks Fallopian tube blockages.

- **Pelvic exam:** Screens for pelvic inflammatory disease, ovarian cysts and uterine structural issues.

- **Prolactin blood test:** Screens for high levels caused by tumors, hypothyroidism or medications. Inhibits ovulation.

- **Glucose tolerance test:** Assesses insulin resistance associated with irregular periods, especially in PCOS. Checks diabetes risk.

- **Thyroid panel:** Measures TSH, T3, T4, and antibodies related to hypothyroidism or hyperthyroidism which frequently cause abnormal periods.

- **Karyotype blood test:** For genetic issues like Turner's syndrome that lead to premature ovarian failure.

Testing provides the missing puzzle piece so remedies can be tailored.

## Potential Treatment Options

After identifying any underlying causes, your doctor will advise appropriate treatment which may involve:

**Medications:** Such as birth control pills, ovulation induction drugs, thyroid medications, or ovulation suppressants.

**Dietary approaches:** Nutritional therapies and supplements to improve insulin resistance, inflammation, and hormonal health often help normalize cycles.

**Surgery:** To remove uterine fibroids, polyps, cysts, scar tissue or endometriosis lesions which can contribute to abnormal bleeding and cramps.

**Intrauterine devices:** Certain IUDs reduce heavy prolonged bleeding from fibroids and endometriosis.

**Metformin and inositols:** For PCOS patients, these improve insulin sensitivity and reduce androgens allowing more normal ovulation.

**Thyroid treatments:** Hypothyroidism requires thyroid hormone replacement. Hyperthyroidism involves anti-thyroid drugs, radioactive iodine, or surgery. Restoring thyroid function helps menstrual regulation.

**Hormone replacement therapy:** Short-term estrogen/progesterone therapy can reboot ovarian function in some cases but doesn't address the root cause.

**Assisted reproductive technology:** IVF with ICSI can help achieve pregnancy in many cases of irregular periods.

# Medications That Regulate Cycles

If no underlying disorder is found, medications that directly prompt ovulation, trigger withdrawal bleeding, or suppress ovulation can override cycle irregularities:

**Estrogen therapy:** Restarts periods in women who don't ovulate due to low body weight or hypothalamic amenorrhea. Also prescribed for post-pill amenorrhea.

**Provera (progesterone):** Induces a bleed when periods have been absent for a prolonged time, especially helpful for amenorrhea.

**Oral contraceptives:** The pill regulates bleeding and suppresses ovulation. Allows you to schedule a bleed by taking placebo pills. Often prescribed for irregular cycles without a clear pathology.

**Ovulation induction medications:** Like clomiphene citrate help stimulate ovaries to release mature eggs in anovulatory cycles. Must be carefully monitored.

**Gonadotropin injections:** More potent fertility drugs containing FSH, LH, or hCG can trigger ovulation when oral medications fail.

**GnRH analogs:** Synthetic hormones that first flare up then suppress ovarian function. Useful for conditions like endometriosis.

Discuss medication risks, side effects, dosage instructions, and fertility implications with your doctor to make an informed choice.

# When to Consider IVF

For women desiring pregnancy, severely irregular cycles, absent ovulation, blocked tubes, or unresponsive thin uterine lining may necessitate in vitro fertilization with ICSI to achieve conceive:

**Irregular Cycles:** Makes conception difficult by creating uncertainty around ovulation timing. IVF controls follicle development and isolates the optimal time for embryo transfer.

**Anovulatory Cycles:** Without ovulation, pregnancy can't occur naturally. IVF allows egg retrieval and fertilization outside the ovaries.

**Damaged Fallopian Tubes:** Blockages keep sperm from reaching the egg. IVF bypasses the tubes entirely.

**Thin Endometrial Lining:** Too little uterine lining precludes implantation. Some linings thicken better with IVF hormonal preparations.

**Unexplained Infertility:** After testing reveals no clear diagnosis, moving to IVF offers the highest conception success rate.

**Donor Eggs:** For poor egg quality due to advanced age or premature ovarian failure, donor eggs maximize IVF outcomes.

If you're under 35 with irregular cycles impacting fertility, first consider less invasive ovulation induction medications which may suffice. But IVF success rates are highest in your late 20s and early 30s, so don't delay too long if ovulation drugs fail.

---

Seeking a doctor's expertise provides the best opportunity to identify any underlying disorders contributing to abnormal cycles so they can be treated effectively. Testing combined with the right medical and lifestyle interventions helps restore your natural rhythms.

# Chapter 6: Beyond the Period - Improving Your Fertility

Once you've regulated your menstrual cycles, optimizing fertility is the next step if pregnancy is desired. Understanding your personal patterns of ovulation, tracking fertile signs diligently, and engaging in well-timed intercourse can vastly improve your conception chances.

In this chapter, we'll explore:

- Predicting ovulation day

- Extending the fertile window

- Maximizing intercourse timing

- Sperm health factors

- Improving egg quality

- Dealing with luteal phase issues

- When to seek help

Get to know your body's rhythms and amplify your efforts during peak fertility for the highest probability of conceiving naturally.

## Predicting Ovulation

Pinpointing your likely ovulation date each cycle is key to pregnancy achievement. Watch for:

**Ovulation pain:** Some women experience a dull ache or twinge near the ovaries around ovulation due to fluid or blood leaking from the rupturing follicle.

**Cervical fluid changes:** Fluid becomes clear, slippery, and stretchy at ovulation – resembling raw egg whites. This supports sperm motility.

**BBT dip:** Your basal body temperature drops .5-1 °F 1-2 days before your LH surge triggers ovulation.

**Positive OPK test:** Home urine ovulation predictor kits detect your LH surge 24-48 hours before ovulation. Test daily leading up to expected ovulation.

**Mittelschmerz:** Around ovulation, some women feel a sharp ovarian pinching sensation lasting a few minutes due to follicle rupture.

**Breast tenderness:** Swelling and soreness of the breasts sometimes emerges just before ovulation due to rising estrogen levels.

**Sex drive changes:** Many women experience heightened libido and sexual arousal around the fertile window.

Pinpointing ovulation day accurately helps focus fertility efforts at the optimal time.

# Extend the Fertile Window

The 6 days spanning the 5 days before ovulation and ovulation day itself mark your prime fertile window each cycle. Some studies suggest the window may be broader– up to 10 days– due to sperm lifespan.

Maximize chances by having intercourse every 2-3 days starting soon after your period ends up until ovulation:

- Sperm can survive 3-5 days inside you, so they are ready to fertilize the egg after ovulation.

- However, the most fertile mucus occurs 1-2 days before ovulation.

- More frequent sex when fertile cervical fluid is present just before ovulation ensures fresh sperm is ready to capitalize on the egg release.

- Visual cues like slippery mucus and positive OPKs indicate ovulation is approaching – increase frequency.

Don't just rely on ovulation day. Instead, cover the full fertile window by:

- Tracking your cycles for a few months to establish pattern

- Starting sex before estimated ovulation

- Noting mucus and OPK cues of impending ovulation

- Increasing intercourse when you see signs ovulation is nearing

# Maximize Intercourse Timing

When trying to conceive, proper timing of intercourse around ovulation reaps benefits:

- Strive for every other day during the fertile window. Daily is too frequent.

- The 1-2 days before ovulation are most critical as cervical fluid nourishes sperm and ovary prepares to release egg.

- Ovulation day remains important to catch the egg. But ovulation is harder to time exactly.

- The 1-2 days after ovulation still offer some chance as the egg can survive for 12-24 hours.

- Have sex in the morning when sperm counts tend to be highest if possible.

- Avoid lubricants as they can impede sperm motility. Optimal fertile cervical fluid already lubricates.

- If sexual frequency declines in your relationship, be intentional about setting aside time for sex during peak fertile days.

Staying engaged frequently in the build-up to ovulation, then directly hitting the ovulation day optimizes the probability of conception each cycle.

## Support Your Partner's Fertility

Up to 50% of fertility challenges involve male factor issues like low sperm count or motility. Tips to improve sperm:

**Limit alcohol:** Chronic drinking is associated with decreased sperm count and abnormal sperm shape impacting fertility.

**Quit smoking:** Cigarette toxins reduce sperm count. Marijuana impacts sperm health and ovulation.

**Minimize stress:** High stress also lowers sperm count and motility. Cortisol impairs testosterone needed for sperm production.

**Avoid tight underwear:** Tighter briefs or underwear create scrotal heat that can reduce sperm count and quality.

**Get checked for varicocele:** Varicose veins around the testicle cause overheating which damages sperm. Treatments can help.

**Take supplements:** Zinc, selenium, Vitamin C, and L-arginine all support healthy sperm production and development.

**Exercise moderately:** Regular cardio activity improves testosterone levels and blood flow needed for sperm development. But excessive exercise is detrimental.

**Eat antioxidant foods:** Fruits, vegetables, nuts and whole grains provide antioxidants that improve sperm quality and protect sperm DNA.

His sperm health impacts fertility as much as your cycle health. Work together to create optimal conditions.

## Improve Egg Quality

Diminished ovarian reserve and poor egg quality make conception less likely as we age. You can enhance egg quality through strategies like:

**Take CoQ10:** Required for egg metabolism. Doses of 600-800mg daily improve egg quality and embryo development. Start several months before trying to conceive.

**Acupuncture:** Increases blood flow to ovaries and uterus. Shown to reduce chromosomal abnormalities in eggs which raises IVF success rates.

**Eat organic and avoid BPA:** Pesticides and plastics with BPA cause egg DNA damage. Choosing organic foods and avoiding packaged items in plastic minimizes exposure.

**Make sleep a priority:** Chronic sleep deprivation and disruption of circadian rhythms is associated with reduced ovarian reserve markers and poorer IVF outcomes.

**Manage stress:** High cortisol from chronic stress impairs ovarian response and lowers egg quality. Stress reduction protects eggs.

**Maintain normal weight:** Being over- or underweight leads to more immature and anomalous eggs due to the effects of insulin resistance and inflammation on follicular development.

**Limit strenuous exercise:** Excessive aerobics stresses the ovaries. Weightlifting is fine.

Protecting your precious eggs from harm ensures the highest quality eggs possible each cycle.

# Address Luteal Phase Defects

A luteal phase spanning less than 10 days prevents adequate progesterone levels and endometrial thickening needed to implant the fertilized egg. Causes include:

- Premature drop in progesterone

- Low progesterone production

- Uterine contractions before implantation is complete

- Poor endometrial receptivity

If you notice premenstrual spotting or a shorter cycle length, get your progesterone tested 7 days after ovulation. Levels below 10 ng/ml indicate a deficiency requiring treatment such as:

- Progesterone supplements

- Progesterone-releasing IUD

- Supplements to lengthen the luteal phase like vitamin B6

- IVF with hormone medications to ensure thicker lining

Don't ignore mid-luteal phase spotting if you are trying to conceive. Get it addressed promptly to help implantation succeed.

# Seeking Fertility Help

If well-timed intercourse for 6 months fails to achieve pregnancy under age 35, or after 3-4 months over age 35, seek fertility testing to uncover any issues. Evaluation might include:

- Bloodwork to test hormone levels

- Ultrasound to examine uterine lining thickness after ovulation

- Post-coital testing to assess sperm motility and cervical mucus

- Laparoscopy to check for structural problems like endometriosis

- Semen analysis to assess sperm health parameters

- Hysteroscopy to look for uterine abnormalities

Treatment options for fertility challenges include:

- Ovulation induction medications to stimulate ovulation

- Intrauterine insemination (IUI) to enhance sperm numbers in the uterus

- Surgery to remove endometriosis lesions or fibroids

- IVF with or without ICSI to achieve fertilization when IUI fails

- Donor eggs or sperm when indicated

Seeking help sooner for any suspected fertility issues improves your odds of success faster.

While regulating your cycles is the vital first step, tailored strategies to leverage your window of peak fertility each month lead to the highest chances of conception. Monitoring fertility signs, supporting egg and sperm health, and resolving luteal phase issues cultivates optimal circumstances for new life to take root and flourish.

# Conclusion

Restoring regular menstrual cycles empowers you to reclaim balance and fertility. While the path demands patience and self-compassion, you now have a comprehensive guidebook equipping you to decode your body's messages, identify underlying issues, and implement tailored solutions to revive your rhythmic flow.

We've covered powerful lifestyle remedies within your control including:

- Adopting a menstrual-friendly diet to balance hormones

- Reducing stress and anxiety to inhibit cortisol

- Achieving more restorative sleep to align with circadian rhythms

- Balancing exercise with adequate fuel for your body

- Minimizing toxic exposures that disrupt endocrine function

You've also learned about natural therapies that gently coax your body back into harmony:

- Targeted herbs and supplements to optimize hormonal balance

- Essential oils that relieve menstrual symptoms

- Traditional Chinese Medicine and acupuncture techniques

- Ayurvedic approaches to reduce inflammation

Most importantly, you understand when medical guidance is prudent to uncover and address any underlying conditions perpetuating irregular menstruation. With testing and evidence-based treatments, lasting regulation can be attained.

Armed with a nuanced comprehension of your menstrual physiology, you can now chart your fertility signals, pinpoint ovulation, support cycle health through nutrition and self-care, and lean into your window of peak monthly conception potential if pregnancy is desired.

Yet appreciate that restoring natural rhythms requires an intuitive, whole-person approach. Be patient and tender with your body's process. Track subtle changes sessionally, not daily. Progress happens in gradual waves, not liner steps. Keep the faith through setbacks.

Your menstrual cycle provides a vital feedback loop reflecting your overall health. Learning its messages allows you to be proactive about your wellbeing.

Now you have the resources and self-advocacy skills to understand your unique menstrual language. Stay attuned to what your body is whispering and guide it back into harmonic flow.

Whenever your cycles grow irregular, return to this book's wisdom. Within these pages you'll always find support, insight and pathways forward.

Keep shining your compassionate awareness on your embodied experience. With time, your hormones will respond and your cycle will revert back to its natural state of balance.

Trust in your body's innate wisdom to find its way home. You've got this! One small step at a time, your vitality and rhythm can be restored.

# About the Author

As a naturopathic doctor and certified health coach, Omolola Habib is devoted to supporting women on their journey to restore hormonal balance and menstrual health.

After years struggling with her own irregular cycles, Omolola was driven to find answers through natural medicine when conventional treatments failed her. She dove deep into the study of naturopathy, nutrition, and women's health.

Today, Omolola skillfully blending naturopathic therapies with lifestyle medicine to guide women toward hormonal harmony. She takes an holistic approach focused on uncovering the root causes of cycle irregularities unique to each woman.

Omolola is known for her warmth and compassion. She believes deep listening allows the body's wisdom to reveal the path forward. Her personal experience with menstrual issues fuels her passion to empower other women to reclaim their natural rhythms.

As a clinician, researcher, and educator, Omolola draws on extensive expertise. But she makes complex topics relatable and actionable. Her book, Getting Your Cycle Back on Track, condenses her wisdom into an accessible guide to support women on their journey toward menstrual wellbeing and fertility.